PRACTICAL CHANGE

8 Ways to Rejuvenate Your Life

Noelle Federico
with J. Allan Jones

Music City News Publishing Inc.
1616 Westgate Circle
Brentwood, TN, 37027

www.practicalchanges.com

For information or permissions write:
Music City News Publishing Inc.
1616 Westgate Circle
Brentwood, TN 37027

FIRST EDITION

Cover Design by Steve Linde

Excerpts from Seasons of Prosperity, Is Money the Matter,
Bridging The Gaps and A Tonic for the Mind
used with permission from
Toni Stone, Wonderworks Studio.

ISBN # 0-9768737-0-2

Library of Congress # 2005904118

PRACTICAL CHANGE –

Dedication

To God with whom all things are possible...

To my Mother, my first and best teacher, you are forever an inspiration...I carry your heart in my heart and I love you.

To the memory of Antonio T. Federico, who is my hero...and to Antonio M. Federico who is my joy.

To the Greatest Love of My Life, you have truly taught me what it is to love unconditionally and without reservation. My world is always brighter when you are close at hand, I carry your soul in my heart and I thank you for everything past, present and future.
I LOVE YOU.

With Great Gratitude, I Acknowledge these people...

My son, Antonio, who inspires me and moves me forward everyday.

My Mother, Toni Stone, who is the most incredible woman I know.

My father, Lee Acker, who has reminded me how important each moment is. Thanks for being my Dad and for being a part of our lives.

My Stepfather, Steve Overton, who is a living Saint, Thank you for all that you do. You are a good man.

My Grandmother, Alice/Elizabeth, who truly taught me to serve other people first, you have always been the Light of my life and I love you.

My family~ Uncle Mike, always there and always my champion; Uncle Rich, the Ultimate Godfather and my Superhero when I was a little girl; Karen, the Best Girl; Rick, Auntie Polly, Auntie Peggy and Tony... you have always believed in me and you have taught me what love is.

My very best friend and one of the most brilliant and compassionate souls I have ever met, Jeff Jones ~ without you none of this would be. Your friendship and love enrich my life daily beyond measure — my love and gratitude to you always.

My closet companions without whom my life would be meaningless: Faeda (Lucy) who adds laughter to my world, my Superhero Steve Gill, my BIG brother Gerard, you are the BEST. Mark Bryn, the strong, silent force of love in my life. Erin, who has truly been a GIFT FROM GOD~without you nothing would get done, you are a treasure... Marty Lotito, you have proven to be my personal fitness inspiration and an excellent friend,

Suzanne L., Tina J, Justin, Scottie, Suz and Bryan Jasper, Steve Linde. Thank you for everyway you help me and for everything that you do for me... I truly, truly LOVE YOU ALL.

All of the people that help us all of the time: Kathy, Gordon, Diana, Jane S., Serban and Dragos, Dr. Gephardt, Mike and Ginny D., Ginny, Bill, Cyndi, Diane, Star, Kat A.- the world's greatest publicist, Manny, Marvis and the staff at World's Gym in Tn., Keith and Susan from Donelson and their staff, Kathy Bennett and the Reeves-Sain crew, the Cumulus staff, and the Radio America crew.

My friends from forever- Dr. Shirley Crandall who started all this, Christine, Wayne, Rodney, Chuck, David, Jeff L., Kristine, Mara, JDK, Paul, Steve, Jenny, Toni and Tom, Michael S., Gifford, Deb S., Janice, Roberta, and Markey — you all helped make me what and who I am.

Thank you to all our Nature's Youth customers, distributors and retailers... thank you for allowing us to make a difference in your lives.

May God prosper and bless you always.

Jeff Would Like to Thank...

- Dolores for her love

- His Grandfather, Orin, for always being there

- Steve, Eric and Celeste for their love and devotion

- Dr. Henry N. Peters for his love and guidance

- Michelle, Ashley, Brooke, Connor and Bill for their continued love and support.

- Noelle for her continued devotion

- G. Gordon Liddy for his friendship and support of Nature's Youth

- Diana K. for all that you have done to support us

- Dragos and Serban, his good buddies, for always being there and for their friendship and support

- The other G-Man for his friendship and support

- And all of the people that have inspired me along the way.

PRACTICAL CHANGE –

PRACTICAL CHANGE
8 Ways to Rejuvenate Your Life

Table of Contents

PRACTICAL CHANGE –

"Whatever you can do
or dream you can,
begin it.

Boldness has genius,
power and magic
in it.
Begin it now."

~ Goethe

Introduction

I've changed, I used to be fat and now I'm not. I used to eat sugar and now I don't. I used to think that pondering about good health was better left to the 'earthy, crunchy' people and now I know that it is something our whole culture needs to concern themselves with.

I'm not a Holy Roller nor am I a fitness expert, I am a real person who lost 60 pounds and changed my life and my thinking as a result. The weight stayed off and the changes have caused me to reinvent myself. I am now the Vice President of a Nutritional Supplement company called Nature's Youth and for the past three years I have become increasingly more alarmed at the rising rates of overweight Americans and the overall decline of good health. It seems to me that we have become a society that has given itself permission to be unhealthy, because being healthy is far too much work. Its true, being healthy, exercising, eating correctly and taking the time to take care of yourself is a lot of work. However, being sick and fat will also be a lot of work, not to mention you will have a far shorter lifespan.

To change is uncomfortable and it requires hard work and a commitment from you to yourself.

We live in a society that would have us believe that weight loss can be achieved with little effort by taking a special pill or staying on the latest fad diet for a few short weeks. As my friend Steve Gill says, "The truth hurts, feel the pain." The truth in this case being that sustained weight loss and good health require permanent lifestyle changes that are often difficult.

This book has been designed to give you educational information and provide some new ideas to inspire you.

I am a single, working mother and if I can change my life, so can you. Staying healthy is a work in progress and everyday I have the opportunity to work on myself, set higher goals and maintain my weight loss. Everyday the choice is mine and some days I eat potato chips and pizza and some days I skip the treadmill and everyday I drink Lattes from Starbucks...most days I make smart choices and most days I workout and I'm in the best shape of my life, so it's paid off. Please note that there has not been one day in three years that I have run overjoyed to the treadmill, everyday I have to remind myself of my commitment to be healthy and exercise and some days I have to call on someone else to remind me. Support systems are a blessing...

Have a little faith in you, I do, you're worth it and I know that you can attain your goals if you make an effort. I will intend that you are enlivened by reading the pages of this book and that something in here causes you to take action for change.

The contents are presented in an "easy read" fashion with 8 ways to rejuvenate your life. Webster's defines rejuvenate as: to make young again, to restore, to uplift, to make fresh.

In addition to the suggestions, we have provided a commentary at the end of each chapter. The founder of Nature's Youth, Jeff Jones, has been kind enough to share his thoughts with you at the end of each section. Jeff has some great insights on the nutrition/health industry and what it takes to be a success.

Enjoy and thank you for taking the time to read this.

PRACTICAL CHANGE –

Prologue

Milton Erickson said, "Change will lead to insight far more often than insight will lead to change." Every change in my life has taught me something about myself and every change in my life has made me uncomfortable in some way. Change is designed to shake us up so that new things can be created. Change is both challenging and powerful. The very nature of change breathes new life into us; it has us sitting on the edge of our seats straining to see what's next.

This book talks about getting healthy, more importantly; it talks about what it takes to enact change in your life. Everyone can benefit from some type of change as it fosters growth in human beings.

Workable, lasting change starts with telling yourself the truth about what isn't working and then taking practical steps to do things differently.

In my experience, I have discovered 8 important factors that contribute to lasting change. Those 8 factors make up the 8 ways to rejuvenate your life referenced in the title. I believe that all 8 factors are equally important in regards to incorporating lasting change into your life.

While reading this book I invite you to start an investigation into your own life to determine what changes are necessary to create a desirable future.

**The power to create the future
lies within you...*USE IT WISELY***

Some helpful thoughts to have...

Affirmations taken from <u>Seasons of Prosperity</u> by Toni Stone

- I recognize and release resistance to changing
- I realize that to do things the way I've always done them is to stay the same
- I have the idea of changing...
  I am willing to start changing
- I am able to have and receive new directions
- I am living immediately without previous limits...
  no limits allowed, no limits exist!
- I follow new directions fearlessly to produce changes
- No longer am I hesitant taking on risk...
  I recognize stops, they disappear.
- My vision reveals what's next for me...
  I am exuberant.
- I complete what's been, and move
  to what's not yet been...
- Resistance dissolved...enthusiasm has replaced it...
- Endings create new beginnings,
  forward into the process
- I am ready to receive next directions.
- New directions, create new ideas as seeds for starting.
- I have the idea of changing.
- The processing for what's new has already begun.
- I retain full assurance in all that's falling apart...
- letting go of what's been, is good now, I can be sure.

"Reality is merely an illusion, albeit a persistent one..."
— Albert Einstein

"Reality can be beaten with enough imagination."
— Jules de Gautier

The First Way...
Get A Reality Check

The first part of changing or improving anything is to first determine, honestly, where you are now. We will call this a *'Reality Check'*. Conducting an honest reality check with yourself will help you determine the areas that require change. When conducting a Reality Check it is necessary to be completely honest with yourself. If you feel that you are overweight then step on the scale and see how overweight you truly are.

Reality Checks can be a shock to the system... here's how mine went. A little over three years ago I was at a chiropractor's appointment; I had been going to the same chiropractor for 12 years, so needless to say I considered this woman a friend. At that appointment Dr. Crandall informed me that she believed I was at least 40 pounds overweight! I was appalled, shocked, outraged—after all I was a size 14 which wasn't terrific but in my opinion, I was by no means FAT. I mean a size 14 after you just had a baby was NORMAL, wasn't it. I left her office that day and I was so mad, who was she to tell me that I was fat?

Hint: When something bothers you this much it probably bears looking into.

My Mother has always told me that if someone says something about you and secretly you think its true then it will bother you. She puts it this way, "If someone called you an aardvark and you knew you weren't one then you wouldn't care, however if someone called you an aardvark and secretly you thought you were one then you would be outraged at the comment." So, pondering this counsel from my Mother I determined that in fact, I must be overweight… in other words FAT.

Reality Sets In

Okay, so I have accepted the reality that in fact I weigh too much. The question now becomes what do I do about it? With some coaching from my friends I determine that Weight Watchers (WW) is a good place to start. Being the outspoken Italian that I am, it quickly became apparent to me that I was not a "meeting person". This is largely due to the fact that I have little tolerance for someone weeping that they ate an entire chocolate cake yet they couldn't understand why they hadn't lost weight that week.

Therefore, the Weight Watchers at Home Program became my vehicle of choice. My first day on Weight Watchers consisted of opening a frozen WW meal and quickly deciding that I would starve if this was all I could eat. I called my girlfriend and wanted to know, "where was the rest of the meal?" That day I ate two frozen meals and I just counted the points for both. The good news is now one of those meals fills me up, imagine that?

Counting points became a way of life and I made it into a game. If I worked out more I got to eat more. Good News! I also discovered that our *Nature's Youth*

Diet Lift product stopped my appetite dead in its tracks and that was very beneficial. Diet Lift enabled me to be content with salads for lunch, which are zero points on WW. Zero, if there is no salad dressing involved and I wasn't about to waste precious points on salad dressing, (after all, rabbits don't use salad dressing).

I also decided that my penchant for anything and everything chocolate was not going to serve me well so I gave up all sugar. If I wasn't going to have chocolate nothing sweet would do anyway so why not just go cold turkey. Be advised that I was the biggest fan of Drake's Cakes Devil Dogs and could be found with Nestle Crunches always in my car or purse. I was the Queen of chocolate.

Water and low fat popcorn became my new found friends. I began to examine the entire concept of exercise and nutrition and I discovered that most of us are sadly misinformed when it comes to portion size. A restaurant meal is usually two to three portions of food. This was very interesting news as we Italians are taught to eat everything on our plates because people in other parts of the world are starving. You can quickly figure out that most of us are over consuming simply by eating what is put in front of us. One can also see how this behavior would contribute to 65% of Americans being overweight.

Seeing Results

Within a few months I had dropped to a size 10 and then to an 8 and after about 10 months I was a size 4. If you had told me three years ago that at 5'8" I would ever see size 4, I would have laughed you out of the room. However, size 4 it continues to be, three years later and holding. This proves that change can happen if you are committed enough. I am a living example of sustained weight loss and successful change and you can be too.

The project of weight loss and getting healthy or enacting any kind of lifestyle change is an ongoing one, it is never done, it is never over and you must never become complacent. The changes that you make to lose weight are changes that must become a permanent part of your lifestyle. For instance I used to eat only white bread; if you said 'multi-grain' to me I would stick out my tongue and turn away. Now all I eat is low fat, multi-grain bread except for the occasional Italian loaf at a good restaurant.

Water and popcorn are still my best friends, next to Jeff, Faeda, Steve and Gerard of course. I still take *Diet Lift* before workouts and I am on the treadmill at least 20 minutes a day plus training with a trainer several times a week. It isn't any easier, it has just become part of my routine so it doesn't seem so horrid.

- *Was it worth it?* **Yes.**
- *Does it continue to be worth it?* **Yes.**
- *Do I feel better?* **Yes.**
- *Am I a different person because of the weight loss?* **Yes.**
- *Do I LOVE exercising?* **No.**

A Reality Check For You

I have a friend that said she wanted to lose weight, when I inquired how much weight she wanted to lose she said she didn't know. "Well how much do you weigh?" I asked. "I don't know." she replied. She further went on to say that she did not want to get on the scale because it would make her depressed.

Hint: Avoiding reality is never helpful.

"GET ON THE SCALE!" I advised. She did, then she cried and then she got over it and got started on a plan. As I write this she is 12 pounds lighter and counting.

In order to foster change you must admit to yourself what the problem is. This can often be the most painful part of the whole process. Many of us fool ourselves into thinking that there aren't any issues to deal with, our clothes are tighter but we're not fat, we drink a six pack every night but we're not addicted, we smoke but just when we drink or when we're stressed or depressed or…

Our credit cards are maxed out but we don't have a spending problem, you get the picture. Wake up and get honest with yourself, give yourself a reality check. Once you have determined what the reality is then you can become powerful in the circumstance. If you are lying to yourself the circumstance has power over you. When you tell the truth to yourself you get your power back, that power will enable you to make the changes that are required in your life.

The Consequence of Change

As you become empowered and start taking action to improve your life and your health, you will discover that certain circumstances, people, places and things may no longer suit you. Things in your life that are resistant to change will need to fall away in order for you to achieve your goals—sometimes this includes people. There will be people in your life that refuse to engage in their own *'Reality Check'* and therefore will be unable to support yours. I lost a few friends when I lost weight and changed my lifestyle; I suddenly became the enemy as I no longer wanted to spend time complaining about my plight in life. I have been called too skinny, anorexic, bony and even likened to a Purdue chicken (not the Oven Stuffer Roaster). Although this has hurt my feelings, I'm smart enough to know that some people don't have the drive to change so they need to knock down anyone around them that does.

Hint: People that insult you and make fun of your efforts to change are NOT your friends.

Stay focused on your goals and when people have something unkind to say smile and thank them for sharing and then get away from them FAST. Help like that you don't need. Surround yourself with people and circumstances that will support your wish to change; we'll talk more about that in Chapter 5.

Change has a natural way of clearing a path for itself. When you commit yourself to change, life will naturally begin to move obstacles out of your way. Your job is to allow the obstacles to be removed, don't try to hang on to people and things that no longer serve you. It will quickly become clear to you what needs to be eliminated from your life. Trust this process and know that for everything that moves out something better is moving in.

So take off your Rose colored glasses, conduct your *'Reality Check'* and get ready to formulate a plan of action.

And Jeff Says...

In life I've discovered that changes have to be taken in small steps.

In order to go through the process of change you have to be honest with yourself and identify the areas in your life that need to be changed in order of importance. Before this can take place you have to inventory your present life situation and remove the obstacles that could prevent positive change.

These obstacles can be a number of different things, like: continued bad habits, friends that inhibit your success, mental blocks, lack of desire and low self-esteem.

Once you have listed your obstacles start to remove them from your present life situations. This will enable your path to success to become clearer.

About Winning

Affirmations taken from <u>Seasons Of Prosperity</u> by Toni Stone

- I am winning now
- I am truly motivated
- I push through all barriers as a natural winner
- I do what produces results each day
- I know what to do and I do it
- I am inspired from within
- I have resources to keep motivated
- I have productive communication skills
- I have courage to do what works over and over again
- When people don't like what I do it's okay with me
- I keep on no matter what happens
- I keep on doing what needs to be done
- I am no longer stopped by invalidation
- I image what I want and live from those pictures
- I am successful and so are the people around me
- Success is a process; I am in it, I keep on
- I am a natural winner

"A dream becomes a goal when action is taken toward its achievement."
— Bo Bennett

"To accomplish great things, we must not only act, but also dream; not only plan, but also believe."
— Anatole France

The Second Way...
Take Action: Formulate the Master Plan

With the results of your **Reality Check** in hand it's time to get into action. First a goal is required, based on what you have discovered about yourself, what is it that you most want to change? If weight loss is your issue a tiered goal system is best with losing 10% of your body weight being the first desired result. Research has shown that the best way to achieve lasting weight loss is by losing 2~3 pounds per week. If smoking is your issue perhaps cutting down to half would be a good first goal. The idea here is to invent realistic goals that can be achieved with some effort on your part. It is not going to make you feel like a success if you set crazy goals that are unlikely to be attained. For instance, if you are an inherently LAZY person that loves to lie on the couch and now you want to become fit, promising yourself a trip to the gym everyday is not wise. You would be better served by making a commitment to get to the gym 3 days a week. Once you accomplish that and have made those trips to the gym a routine you can come from a place of success and set a higher goal. Even 10 minutes of exercise a day is better than nothing.

My first goal was to lose 10% of my total body weight, which was about 18 pounds. In order to make this happen I determined that counting points needed to be supplemented with the dreaded 'physical activity'. Walking seemed to be the easiest way to incorporate exercise into my life. At the beginning I didn't have the means to join a gym or hire a personal trainer. It was only after three years of hard work that I decided a trainer was required to take me to the next fitness level.

Do not be fooled into thinking that just because I've lost weight I love to exercise. If you ask Marty (my personal trainer), he will tell you that although I may be his most lovable client I am also his biggest whiner. A workout with me consists of me whining and complaining and Marty patiently instructing—this hasn't changed in 6 months. Clearly, Marty is a saint to put up with me since when I'm irritated I am very unpleasant. Marty's support has also gotten results as I am now toned and have less body fat, plus we continue to set new goals. My current goal is to have magazine quality, FLAT ABS in two months. Marty and I are working on that one!!!!

Now, if I weighed 350 pounds, striving for magazine quality abs in 2 months time would be an unrealistic goal that would only serve to make me feel bad when I couldn't attain it.

When setting your personal goals take into account your current attitudes, circumstances and behaviors. Try to set goals that will work into your life without an incredible amount of effort. Be realistic about what you expect from yourself and take an inventory on what hasn't worked for you in the past.

Hint: If it didn't work for you in the past, you can be pretty sure it won't work now. Try something NEW.

Take heed of the definition of *INSANITY*: *Doing the same thing over and over again and expecting a different result.*

Invest in a special notebook and use it to write down your goals, if you can't write them you certainly can't expect to manifest them.

Get Into Action

Every goal needs an action plan to accompany it. The action plan is where you break down how that goal is going to manifest, without the action plan your goal is merely an airy, fairy wish. And airy, fairy wishes are more effective in children's stories. I suggest that in your notebook you write your goals and then make at least 5 action steps to back up each goal.

Example:

Goals
1. Lose 18 pounds in 9 weeks

Actions
- Join Weight Watchers and count points
- Drink 8 glasses of water per day
- Cut out sweets
- Walk at least 20 min. 3 x per week
- Paste sexy women in bathing suits to refrigerator for inspiration
- Start using a WW cookbook for food ideas

Writing all this down will make it easier for you to be accountable to yourself and others. Change is work and needs to be treated as such, it will not just occur without an effort on your part.

Once you have clearly defined your goals and the actions required to make them happen, it's easier to determine how to fit new behaviors into your life. If you know that you need to get to the gym three times a week then you can plan your schedule accordingly. First of course, find a gym and become a member.

In order to support your efforts of change you need to start learning how to make yourself important. All that stuff you have to do will still be there, all those people that need you to take care of them will still be there. Trust me, you will be a lot more effective in your life if you are being true to yourself first. After all, if you are an overweight, unhealthy, resentful mess how much can you really get done anyway?

Set up your Master Plan so that you are taking some actions everyday toward your goals. Even the smallest steps on a daily basis will assist you in achieving the desired result. If I couldn't make it to the gym, I'd walk around the block and do some sit-ups, sometimes it was only 15 minutes—remember 15 minutes is better than no minutes.

Celebrate Your Successes

Have you noticed that people don't celebrate enough? Celebrate your successes, even the little ones. If you walked away from that chocolate cake, or put out the cigarette or left a shopping cart full of useless items at the check out—Celebrate that, acknowledge yourself, great job, good for you…

Whatever you speak about and think about you will get more of, so spend your time dwelling on what works and what you did right. If you ate the chocolate cake, get over it, move on. The more you suffer over the setbacks the more frequent they will become. Ponder what you want more of, let go of all thoughts that don't support the goal. Be grateful that you have the courage to change and make a big noise for any aspect of changing that occurs. Don't wait for other people to tell you what you have achieved, celebrate yourself, have a party for one. You deserve it!

Put some thought and energy into writing your goals and figuring out what action steps will work for you. Remember to set yourself up for winning by giving yourself goals that you can and will accomplish-small successes will become the foundation for larger ones.

Let's see what Jeff says and then take Nutrition 101.

And Jeff Says...

To be honest with you I am not the greatest planner even though I have great plans...

I've always felt that God has an agenda for me and that it's up to me to enable or activate it on a daily basis. Anyone who knows me well will tell you that although I am thorough I have to remind myself of the details. Therefore, everyday I make a list of things I need to do. My list is comprised of appointments, phone calls to make, daily tasks etc. and it always includes the actions that are necessary to achieve my current goals.

I use my daily list as a goal reminder and I suggest you do the same.

Mix up your choices within each food group

From the U.S. Department of Health and Human Service's booklet, *Finding Your Way to a Healthier You.*
Based on the Dietary Guidelines for Americans, 2005
For more info visit: **www.healthierus.gov/dietaryguidelines**

Focus on Fruits: Eat a variety of fruits-whether fresh, frozen, canned or dried-rather than fruit juice for most of your fruit choices. For a 2,000-calorie diet, you will need 2 cups of fruit each day (for example, 1 small banana, 1 large orange, and a ¼ cup of dried apricots or peaches).

Vary your veggies: Eat more dark green veggies, such as broccoli, kale, and other leafy greens; orange veggies, such as carrots, sweet potatoes, pumpkin, and winter squash; and beans and peas, such as pinto beans, kidney beans, black beans, garbanzo beans, split peas, and lentils.

Get your calcium-rich foods: Get 3 cups of low-fat or fat-free milk-or an equivalent amount of low-fat yogurt and/or low-fat cheese (1 ½ ounces of cheese = 1 cup of milk)—everyday. For kids aged 2 to 8, it's 2 cups of milk. If you don't or can't consume milk, choose lactose-free milk products and/or calcium-fortified foods and beverages.

Make half your grains whole: Eat at least 3 ounces of whole-grain cereals, breads, crackers, rice or pasta everyday. One ounce is about 1 slice of bread, 1 cup of breakfast cereal, or ½ cup of cooked rice or pasta. Look to see that grains such as wheat, rice, oats, or corn are referred to as "whole" in the list of ingredients.

Go lean with protein: Choose lean meats and poultry. Bake it, broil it or grill it. And vary your protein choices—with more fish, beans, peas, nuts and seeds.

Know the limits on fats, salt and sugars: Read the Nutrition Facts label on foods. Look for foods low in saturated fats and trans fats. Choose and prepare foods and beverages with little salt (sodium) and/or added sugars (caloric sweeteners).

"To eat is a necessity, but to eat intelligently is an art."
— La Rochefoucauld

"He that takes medicine and neglects diet, wastes the skill of the physician."
— Chinese Proverb

The Third Way
Take Nutrition 101

Here we are in Nutrition 101, previous to starting Weight Watchers and meeting Jeff I considered nutrition to be something for fitness freaks and granola crunchers. **Webster's defines NUTRITION as:** *being nourished, the series of processes by which an organism takes in and assimilates food for promoting growth and replacing worn or injured tissues, the study of proper balanced diet to promote health.*

If you are anything like me, nutrition no matter what its definition is not something you spend a lot of time thinking about. You basically know that eating 7 chocolate bars in one sitting is bad and that eating a salad has potential health benefits. Color me surprised when I actually started to READ the Nutrition Facts panel on product labels and discovered what we unwittingly consume. Example: Yesterday, my friend Steve Linde and I were talking about this very thing. Steve told me that with the intention of being healthy he had replaced his morning coffee with an Energy drink—thinking of course that the Energy Drink would be the better choice. After arriving at work and consuming the entire bottle, he took a peek at the Nutrition Facts panel and discovered that there were 30 grams of sugar in the drink. Upon closer inspection he further noted that the entire bottle was 2.5 servings!!!! Therefore, he had just consumed 75 grams of sugar, he would have been better off with the coffee.

LESSON— packaging is deceiving, pay close attention to the serving size and the Nutrition Facts panel. There are tons of 'snack size' packages out there that are actually 2 and 3 servings, so if you see the calorie count and miss the serving size you're fooling yourself. Recently I discovered 'snack size' packages of pecans, walnuts and almonds—quickly glancing at the calorie count I noted that one serving was 170 calories. I proceeded to tear open the bag and begin stuffing my face and in a moment of clarity I reviewed the label more carefully and discovered that the bag actually contained 2 servings. Incidentally the bag was SMALL, I mean a handful of nuts and that was 2 servings…for who?? Squirrels!!

Pay attention to what you are putting in your mouth and **_read_** the Nutrition Facts panels (including the ingredients list) on everything. Read the information before you buy the item so that you don't make the same mistake I did with the Fat Free Half and Half—Fat Free Half and Half's first 4 ingredients are all some form of sugar starting with Corn Syrup…that carton of Half and Half got poured down the sink!

Hint: If Corn Syrup, High Fructose Corn Syrup, Fructose or Sugar is one of the first 5 ingredients put it DOWN and WALK AWAY.

A Quick Cholesterol Lesson

In regards to cholesterol know that if you are

overweight this has the potential to negatively effect your cholesterol levels. Your total cholesterol count is made of up of three types: LDL cholesterol (the bad one), VLDL (a mix of triglycerides and cholesterol and HDL (the good one). When you are fat or (overweight for those of us avoiding reality) it creates problems in your body by increasing LDL levels and decreasing HDL levels. The extra weight can also increase triglycerides which is another form of fat in the blood. HDL cholesterol is known as the "good guy" because a high level of it seems to protect against heart trouble. Increased bad cholesterol can lead to clogged arteries which can in turn lead to heart trouble. It's a good idea to have a cholesterol screening done in order to establish what your levels are. Part of acknowledging reality is to establish what the problem areas are, so that you can effectively deal with them.

To successfully manage cholesterol get a screening, lose excess weight, keep away from food high in saturated fats and get going on a regular exercise program. That visit to Kentucky Fried Chicken every week is not worth it. For more information and education on cholesterol visit www.americanheart.org and www.hsph.harvard.edu/nutritionsource/index.html

The Skinny on Carbs

Low Carb-No Carb-Impact Carbs… what does it all mean anyway? The truth is that your body cannot function properly without some carbohydrates as the body breaks down all carbohydrates except fiber and turns them into glucose. Glucose is what the body uses as an energy source. When the body is deprived of carbohydrates (glucose), it has a way of taking the protein out of your muscles, stripping off the nitrogen bits and turning the rest into the glucose it needs. The body will trade muscle for glucose if you deprive yourself of carbohydrates. The bottom line is we need carbs to function properly, so let's talk about what kind and how many.

The Institute of Medicine (IOM) recommends that 45% to 65% of your daily calories come from carbohydrates which break down to a minimum of 130 grams per day. Consuming less than 130 grams of carbs per day will cause your body to start breaking down muscle to get glucose.

When you eat carbohydrates your digestive system is trained to break them down into sugar molecules and convert them to glucose, the body's main source of energy. How fast a carbohydrate is converted has a direct result on your blood sugar. If a carb is converted quickly it causes your blood sugar to spike. Carbs that cause a rapid spike in blood sugar are the ones to stay away from. There is a system for classifying how quickly carbs will be converted by your body; it's called the Glycemic Index (GI). The Glycemic Index is designed to help you determine which carbohydrates will best serve the needs of your body. Carbs with a low GI are optimal and carbs with a high GI should be avoided. Low GI carbs are digested slowly and provide a more subtle change in blood sugar while high GI carbs are digested immediately and cause blood sugar to spike. For example white bread, French fries, soda, bananas and potatoes are all high GI carbs. Most legumes, whole wheat bread, oats, bran and whole fruits are low GI carbs. For a detailed explanation of the GI and to search specific foods visit www.glycemicindex.com.

Hint: If it comes in a box or a bag with a flavor packet throw it away.

When choosing your carbs understand that processed foods, sugar filled snacks, and Soda-Diet or otherwise are all things to AVOID. "Helpful" and "Easy" boxed meal items are only helping us to get fatter as their flavor packets are LOADED with Sodium and a bunch of other unhealthy ingredients. Sodium retains water and can also be found in most carbonated drinks. Read the labels…

Okay, so based on the above information, eat your carbs and be smart about it.

Not All Fats Are Created Equal

The right types of Fat are actually necessary nutrients for the body. Fat supplies essential fatty acids and free fatty acids are the main source of fuel for muscles at rest and during light activity. The stored fat in the body protects vital organs, insulates you from the cold and transports the fat soluble vitamins (A, D, E and K). Stay away from high quantities of Saturated Fat (cheese, butter, meat fat, whole milk) and Trans Fat (fried foods, baked goods, doughnuts, crackers). These are the bad guys.

Polyunsaturated Fats (vegetable oil, margarine) are okay in moderation as they provide vitamin E, however they can sometimes lower HDL cholesterol.

Monounsaturated Fat (poultry, fish, nuts, olive oil) can actually help to lower total cholesterol and Omega-3 Fat (fish, flaxseed) can lower the risk of heart disease. These are the good guys.

A balanced low-fat diet is thought to contain 20% to 35% of calories from fat. The theme in all of this is everything in moderation, to totally deprive your body of any one food group or nutrient is never a good idea.

Hint: A Low~Fat label is not an invitation to eat 9 servings. MODERATION is the key.

A Quick Word About Protein

Protein is responsible for about 75% of your total weight. Protein is in your hair, skin, nails, bones and just about every other part of your body. Since there are about 10,000 different proteins that contribute to who and what you are, protein is obviously pretty important stuff. Amino acids are the building blocks for protein and the body needs a daily supply of amino acids to continue to create the new protein it requires.

Protein needs to be an integral part of your balanced diet and a good mix of proteins is the best plan of attack. Protein always comes packaged with something so make wise choices about your protein sources. For example, a steak can be a great source of protein, however, if it is not a very lean cut it can also contain a good amount of Saturated Fat (one of the Bad Guys).

Some good sources of protein are:

- Any type of nuts
- Lentils
- Kidney Beans
- Split Peas
- Tofu (Yummm!)
- Lean Hamburg
- Chicken
- Tuna

- Fish
- Whole Wheat Bread
- Eggs
- Low Fat Cheddar Cheese
- Low Fat Yogurt
- Broccoli
- Whole Grains

Eat Your Fruits and Veggies, EVERYDAY

Every Diet Plan out there that's worth anything will stress the importance of eating your fruits and veggies on a daily basis. Fruits and Vegetables are filled with all kinds of groovy stuff that will help your body to naturally ward off tons of evil things -heart disease, high blood pressure and cancer to name a few. Those of us who live to count points on WW love these items because they are low points or NO points!!! In fact last week I made the excellent discovery that I could dip celery in salsa and it was ZERO points—so of course I ate an entire package of celery...

The new government Dietary Guideline calls for Americans to eat 5 to 13 servings of fruit and vegetables a day. The truth of the matter is that currently, the average American eats about 3 servings a day. A good goal is about 4.5 cups of fruit and veggies per day. If you can't imagine how you could possibly consume this many servings of fruits and vegetables per day consider drinking a green food supplement like our Youthful Greens product. Drinking a green food supplement will enable you to easily get the required amount of fruits and vegetables on a daily basis.

Hint: French fries ARE NOT a vegetable and the pickles in your fast food sandwich do not constitute a complete serving of vegetables.

Start embracing the fruits and vegetables folks; I can't say enough good things about the benefits of this stuff. Try new things if you tend to get bored with your traditional choices. My favorite thing to do is make a huge pot of what my grandmother calls "garbage soup", which contains all veggies and has a tomato base …the best part, is it has ZERO POINTS.   Be creative and remember that the best way to reap the benefits of fruits and veggies is by consuming a variety of them.

Water, Water Everywhere

Since your body is primarily made up of water it makes perfect sense that you should be consuming a good amount of it everyday. Water helps to re-hydrate your system as well as flush out impurities. I've found that drinking a gallon of water the night before you are going to weigh yourself is also beneficial. The healthy recommendation is 8—8oz. glasses of water a day. I drink at least 6 or 7 bottles a day, the 16.9 fluid ounce size. In fact all you can find in my house to drink is water and coffee, much to the chagrin of any visitors. My advice to everyone who wants to listen is AVOID ALL SODA; I don't care if it's low-carb or Diet… it's not good for you. Sugar filled soda has made a HUGE contribution to the demise of America's good health; it contains empty calories that are good for nothing but a sugar high. Enough said. Increasing your water intake is a vital part of losing weight and staying healthy.

Watch the labels on your water too, as there are companies out there selling filtered water with a design label that makes you think it's from a natural source. It's not that filtered water is bad, just be aware of what you're getting.

> **Product Plug:** *I am happy to report that Nature's Youth is coming out with Natural Spring Water that of course you should try.*

Multi-Vitamins and Other Supplements

In my opinion everyone should be taking a multi-vitamin and given that, Jeff and I have spent a good amount of time formulating what we think is a superior multi-vitamin. I am going to share the information I wrote on **Daily Defense** with you.

What Are Vitamins and Minerals and Why Are They Important?

Vitamins and minerals are nutrients that are essential to life. Vitamins function mostly as coenzymes. Enzymes are catalysts or activators in the chemical reactions that are continually taking place in our bodies. Vitamins are a fundamental part of the enzymes. Enzymes are at the very foundation of all our bodily functions. Without enzymes, you can't breathe, blink, or walk. Your body can't break down proteins into essential amino acids, electrons can't flow, and nerve transmissions can not occur. Minerals, many of which also function as coenzymes, are needed for the proper composition of our body fluids, in blood and bone formation, and to maintain a healthy nerve function. After they have been absorbed, vitamins and minerals actually become part of the structure of the body - of the cells, enzymes, hormones, muscles, blood, and bone.

Who should take Daily Defense?

As most individuals do not eat the variety and quality of foods that would enable them to obtain essential vitamins, minerals and antioxidants, **Daily Defense** is recommended for anyone over 18 years of age.

Why take Daily Defense?

Conceptually we know that good nutrition is essential to our health and well-being, however, the reality is that most of us don't follow a well-balanced diet on a regular basis. *Daily Defense* Multi-vitamins contain anti-oxidants and other nutrients that support your bodily functions, clean your system and help rid your body of "Free Radicals" that build up and can harm your cells, muscles, and organs. Daily Defense formulations also contain enzymes that aid in overall digestion and support your system's ability to absorb nutrients from the foods you do eat.

Now of course there are other multi-vitamins out there besides *Daily Defense* and although I recommend *Daily Defense* (which I named by the way) you can certainly take another multi-vitamin. Make sure that the vitamin you choose has a good list of ingredients as well as a good rate of absorption. For the record- if you got your multi-vitamin at the grocery store it probably isn't doing what you need it to do.

Personally, I supplement my *Daily Defense* with additional calcium as well as a whole host of other items. My daily list: Youthful Greens, Nature's Youth Noni Juice, Garlic, Parsley, Gingko, Echinacea (in the winter months), Zinc, Vitamin C, Flaxseed, Evening Primrose Oil, Coral Calcium, Cayenne Pepper and Vitamin E. My counter is a virtual health food store! Taking all this stuff is a pain, however this year I was able to kick the Flu in three days without any antibiotics.

Bottom Line: Take a good multi-vitamin and supplement it with whatever works for you.

A Health Alert

Those of us over 35 need to be aware of some things that are caused by years of eating a diet heavy in refined carbohydrates such as cereals, muffins, doughnuts, breads, cookies, soda and pasta. A diet like this can cause insulin resistance, high levels of blood fat, weight gain and high blood pressure otherwise known as Syndrome X. These conditions in the body lead to premature aging and can cause an increased risk for heart disease and Type 2 Diabetes.

Some of the symptoms of Syndrome X are feeling tired and mentally sluggish after eating and at other times, having trouble losing extra weight, and elevated blood pressure and cholesterol levels.

Syndrome X can also contribute to free radical damage in the body's cells (oxidation).

Given that Syndrome X is primarily a nutritional disease the best way to reverse its effects and symptoms is by modifying your diet and following a regular exercise program. Diet modification would include drastically reducing consumption of high GI carbs and bulking up on vegetables.

With the knowledge that certain supplements can aid in the reversal of Syndrome X symptoms Jeff developed R-Factors for the Nature's Youth line. R-Factors contains Resveratrol (the stuff in Red Wine) which is a powerful anti-oxidant. It is also a natural compound that appears to boost Sirtuins. Sirtuins are cellular enzymes which appear to be universal regulators of aging in all living organisms. They appear to be guardians of the cell and they allow cells to survive damage. Strengthening the cell's ability to repair itself helps to slow the effects of aging. R-Factors also contains Alpha-lipoic acid which is a powerful anti-oxidant and has been shown to help lower blood sugar levels by increasing insulin sensitivity. Banaba Leaf Extract which has been shown in some human clinical studies to help lower blood sugar in Type 2 diabetes is also part of the R-Factors formulation.

Please be aware of the issues and symptoms of Syndrome X and if you feel that you may be at risk go and consult your doctor or begin to tailor your diet. Remember Syndrome X and Type 2 diabetes can be combated with proper diet and lifestyle changes. So pay attention to what your body is telling you and stop filling it full of high GI carbs.

By the way I have been taking R-Factors for a little over two weeks now and so far I notice that I have more energy and I feel more clear headed when I wake up.

Use Common Sense

Based on what we have just covered you can see that if you use common sense when choosing food you'll be in good shape. Stay away from the bad fats and the high GI carbs, eat lots of veggies, drink your water and grill, bake or broil your meat. Select your calories wisely and eat foods that will support your goals of good health. Stay away from empty calories and watch your sodium intake. Above all READ THOSE LABELS. If you are a constant snacker, try snacking on veggies instead of chips or cookies. Keep fresh fruit around the house and don't put things in your cabinets that you shouldn't be eating. If stuff isn't healthy for you it certainly isn't healthy for the other people in the house.

Well, let's ask Jeff if I covered the topic of nutrition sufficiently and then it's time to talk exercise.

And Jeff Says...

We live in the freest nation in the world. We are free to live life in almost any way we choose. We have the freedom of speech, the freedom of choice, the freedom to vote and the freedom to EAT!

The problem in this country is that we live a life of excess. It's become far to easy to Super Size our meals and in the process we have Super Sized ourselves. With the ability to drive through fast food chains for every meal it's no mystery that 65% of Americans are overweight or obese.

In some way, shape or form nutrition and vitamin supplementation have always been an important part of my life. As a child, I was clinically diagnosed with malnutrition on several occasions and no one knows better than I how economics can effect one's ability to be properly nourished.

Growing up I was determined to have an impact on society in regards to nutrition by developing supplements that would positively effect people's lives. Although I am not a Certified Nutritionist or a Doctor I have studied nutrition for over 22 years and have first hand experience with the benefits of eating well and taking supplements.

It is vitally important that we stay on a life long sensible diet and YES, it's okay to cheat once and awhile...

PRACTICAL CHANGE –

Body-wide Benefits:

A sedentary (inactive) lifestyle increases the chances of becoming overweight and developing a number of chronic diseases. Exercise or regular physical activity helps many of the body's systems function better and keeps a host of diseases at bay. According to the US Surgeon General's report, Physical Activity and Health (1), regular physical activity:

- Improves your chances of living longer and living healthier.

- Helps protect you from developing heart disease or its precursors, high blood pressure and high cholesterol.

- Helps protect you from developing certain cancers, including colon and breast cancer.

- Helps prevent or control type 2 diabetes (what was once called adult-onset diabetes).

- Helps prevent arthritis and may help relieve pain and stiffness in people with this condition.

- Helps prevent the insidious loss of bone known as osteoporosis.

- Reduces the risk of falling among older adults

- Relieves symptoms of depression and anxiety and improves mood

- Controls weight

taken from
http://www.hsph.harvard.edu/nutritionsource/Exercise.htm

PRACTICAL CHANGE –

The human body is made up of some four hundred muscles; evolved through centuries of physical activity. Unless these are used, they will deteriorate.

— Eugene Lyman Fisk

The human body was designed to walk, run or stop; it wasn't built for coasting.

— Cullen Hightower

The Fourth Way...
Put Down the Remote, Get Up and Get Moving

I read somewhere in this month's SELF magazine that the only exercise program that will truly change your body is the one that you will do. I laughed when I read it and I thought to myself, "what a profound truth". You can have the best intentions, the finest equipment, the greatest trainer and the hottest workout gear but if you aren't going to get up off your butt and get to work none of it matters.

The only thing that is going to affect a change in your life is YOU. You have to want it bad enough, you have to be more committed to changing than you are to your current circumstances. Your drive to change and motivate yourself has to be stronger than your wish to be comfortable. The truth of the matter is that change is uncomfortable and change is hard work—real growth as a person comes from the hard work of self-challenge. Change is an inherent part of who we are as human beings, we are meant to be challenged and prevail. Those lessons are what our souls use to grow.

Folks that are 'putting up with' things, conditions,

people and situations that make them unhappy aren't really living; they have lost their zest, zeal and enthusiasm for life. They "put up with" these things because they are afraid of change and its consequences. They are afraid to challenge themselves to find a new way, to do something different, to breakout of the dried-up old thing that has become their life. How many of us wake up each day filled with enthusiasm about what's to come, jumping out of bed because we can't wait to get started. Far too few of us would be my guess…

You and you alone have the power to change your circumstances, your life, your weight, your job, your relationships and your habits. In order to affect change you must be willing to do something different, you need to think differently, speak differently and take new actions.

No matter what areas in your life require change, your attitude will be markedly improved by getting off the couch and doing some sort of physical activity. People that exercise on a regular and consistent basis are known to be healthier and have a more positive attitude.

Keep It Simple

Incorporating physical activity into your life doesn't have to be a huge project; you can make it as simple as adding walking time into your schedule. Optimal results with exercise will occur when it becomes part of your daily routine, much like brushing your teeth or taking a shower. Most of us do certain things everyday without even thinking about them, we just know we need to do them and they are not optional. The easier you can make it for yourself the more likely you are to keep doing it. I've recently discovered that the biggest barrier to a regular exercise program for most people is **TIME**. People seem to feel that they have no **TIME** to fit exercise into their already packed schedules. The problem is that if they do not take the **TIME** to exercise they will end up fitting an unwelcome illness or condition into their schedules. It is actually more desirable to fit an exercise program into your life than an illness. Make **TIME** to exercise.

HINT: The hand to mouth motion of stuffing your face with food is not the kind of exercise we are talking about.

Maintaining good health **IS** worth the time in your schedule. Finding time to exercise is difficult, that is why I am suggesting that you must make it a non-negotiable part of your daily life. Start small, take a daily walk or do a 20 minute exercise video. You need to find something that you like to do and then stick with it. Only you can decide what type of activity will work for you and there are plenty of choices. You can also use Supplements to help you gain the extra boost needed to maintain an exercise program. I highly recommend our *Diet Lift and Nature's Youth RSF* (I have provided brief product information in the Epilogue) as an excellent addition to any good health program. Both of these products will increase your energy and help speed recovery after workouts. *Diet Lift*, as I said earlier, will also reduce your appetite. These products helped and continue to help me immensely.

If you work best with support and structure then join a gym and hire a trainer to get you on track. I love Marty (my trainer) so much that I decided I wanted to help people in the same way he helps me and I am now enrolled in a course to become a Certified Fitness Trainer. By the time we publish this book you will be able to come and train with me at World's Gym in Cool Springs, TN—we'd love to have you workout with us anytime!

In the beginning my exercise program consisted of walking outside and lifting free weights with a Denise Austin weight training tape. That was my program for almost a year as I had no time to get to the gym because my son was an infant. After that first year I purchased a treadmill, a stationary bike and a weight bench and made a gym in the basement. I got poster paper and paints and lined the walls with inspiring phrases like "walk off the weight" and pictures from magazines of people working out. Looking at all that helped me to stay inspired as I still had no time to go to a gym. The point here is that I did what worked for me and because I created a plan that worked with my life, I was able to stay committed to it.

The best advice I can give you…***DO SOMETHING!*** Even 20 minutes a day is better then nothing at all. Take a good look at how your life works and find something to do that will be simple and then fit it into your schedule.

You've Got to Muscle Up

Most people understand the value of cardiovascular exercise, however many people do not understand the equal importance of strength training. This section is designed to help you understand the value of building muscle through strength training.

The Strong Survive... Why you need to strength train.

Strength training is important for young people and even more important for older folks.

Starting in their late 30's or early 40's, most people lose about a quarter pound of muscle every year. By the time they're 80, they've typically lost about a third of their muscle mass. Some of the loss is due to the aging process and some can actually be due to poor nutrition and lack of physical activity.

Muscle is the main ingredient for being healthy, vital and independent as we grow older. It keeps us strong and able to move. It pulls on bone to help bone stay stronger. And it burns more calories than fat burns. Muscle and lean body mass are the metabolic engines in your body. An increase of muscle means your metabolic rate rises, which makes it easier to stay fit. Muscle is also where most of our blood sugar (glucose) goes. When the body breaks down food to make glucose the glucose goes into the bloodstream and most of it gets deposited in the muscle as stored glycogen.

Working to build more muscle can mean lower blood sugar. This can help to ward off the possibility of Type 2 Diabetes. These days we're seeing an epidemic of Type 2 Diabetes because people have unconscious eating habits and they are not actively using their muscles. When muscles aren't in use their cells become resistant to the insulin that the pancreas secretes. This means that the insulin doesn't do what it needs to. If muscle cells are insulin resistant, there is a higher risk of heart disease. And if resistance leads to more glucose in the bloodstream, that can cause Diabetes.

- Strength Training lowers the risk of many chronic diseases
- Evidence suggests that strength training can prevent bone fractures
- Two to three sessions per week of strength training is optimal, lasting 30 to 45 minutes
- You should do six to ten different exercises per session with at least 2 sets of reps
- 30 to 60 minutes of aerobic activity most days of the week is also suggested

Make An Effort

As I said in the Introduction, my wish is that something in here will inspire you enough that you make an effort to change and will do some type of exercise. I would love to be able to magically impart to you all that I have learned so far in this process. The process has been difficult; I have been and continue to be challenged, I have learned and continue to learn about myself. I still have days where I don't exercise and I still have to make a real effort to discipline myself, however the benefits are worth it. I feel better, I look better and I like myself more.

One thing that has really helped me with exercise is keeping an exercise journal. In the exercise journal you keep track of what you do each day and if you do nothing you write that too. I do one journal for each six month period and on bad days I look back in the journal and I get to see how far I've come. Keeping the journals has helped me to acknowledge and celebrate my progress. It has also helped me to see that a bad day or a bad week doesn't last forever. I highly recommend **_The Ultimate Workout Log_ by Suzanne Schlosberg**, *www.houghtonmifflinbooks.com*, as this is the journal I have used for 3 years now and it really helps me stay on track.

A new behavior becomes a habit after 21 days, so if you can make it through the first 3 weeks with your new routine it will then become a part of your life. The good news is that after a period of exercising on a consistent basis your body will actually begin to crave the physical activity. This is a benefit because on the days you don't feel like doing it your body will actually push you to get moving.

Do the best you can and remember that some kind of exercise is better than no exercise at all. Time to ask Jeff for his infinite wisdom....

And Jeff Says...

Based on personal experience I know that starting an exercise program and sticking with it can be difficult. There are often times when business trips or projects interfere with my best intentions to stay healthy. When this happens it is important for me to eat healthy and continue taking my vitamins. The conscious effort of eating healthy and taking vitamins makes it easier for me to jump back on the exercise track as soon as my schedule allows.

Another way I keep my exercise goals alive is, I pay my trainer even when circumstances force me to miss a session. Needless to say I don't miss many.

I have found that it is easier to begin an exercise program with a buddy. Having a friend to workout with can keep you both motivated and supported.

I could not fit my exercise program into my life, so I had to wrap my life around my exercise program and my goals for good health. Making the circumstances of my life work around what I need to do to keep healthy has taken some practice; however, it has ensured that there is always time for exercise.

If you feel that you lack the time to devote to being healthy, I suggest that you evaluate your life and figure out how to fit it in. If I can do it, so can you.

"This is the true joy in life,
the being used for a purpose
recognized by yourself as a mighty one;
the being a force of nature instead of
a feverish, selfish little clod of
ailments and grievances complaining
that the world will not devote itself to
making you happy.

I am of the opinion that my life belongs
to the whole community, and as long
as I live it is my privilege to do for it
whatever I can.

I want to be thoroughly used up when I
die, for the harder I work the more I live.
I rejoice in life for its own sake. Life is
no "brief candle" for me. It is a sort of
splendid torch which I have got hold of
for the moment, and I want to make it
burn as brightly as possible before
handing it on to future generations."

— George Bernard Shaw

"There is no greater Joy nor greater reward than to Make A Difference in someone's LIFE..."
— Sr. Mary Rose McGeady

"Blessed are the poor in spirit: for theirs is the kingdom of heaven. Blessed are they that mourn: for they shall be comforted. Blessed are the meek: for they shall inherit the earth. Blessed are they which do hunger and thirst after righteousness: for they shall be filled. Blessed are the merciful: for they shall obtain mercy. Blessed are the pure in heart: for they shall see God. Blessed are the peacemakers: for they shall be called the children of God.
— Matthew 5:3-9

The Fifth Way...
Look Outside Yourself, Stay Committed, Practice Discipline and Get Support

Whenever I am suffering immensely I immediately begin to look outside myself to see where and whom I can contribute to. No matter what our personal problems are there is always someone out there that can benefit from being contributed to. The finest lesson my family has taught me is how to serve others, as it is by serving others that my life gets made.

When you are feeling blue and overwhelmed by the prospect of the work that lies ahead of you, there is nothing that will restore your soul more then doing something for someone else. Service to others can show up in so many ways: a conversation with a sad friend, sending flowers, sending a card, making cookies, giving a hug, saying 'I Love You', mowing a lawn, visiting an elderly friend, baking a pie, paying for the person's coffee behind you, etc. These small acts of generosity will come back to bless the giver over and over again.

There is always someone with a bigger problem then you, perhaps they are unhealthier or they weigh more or they smoke or they are depressed, whatever their issue is they can certainly benefit from your unconditional acts of generosity. True giving is done with no expectations of reciprocation. Generous people give and serve others because they understand how much it contributes to their own lives. Engaging in self-change is an uncomfortable and difficult task, however, if you look outside yourself and strive to contribute to others your tasks will become easier to bear. In helping other people to achieve good health I find that I will push myself harder so that I can be inspiring to others. There have been many days that I have exercised simply because I knew that to help others I had to stay on track.

Look Around You

Strive to be the kind of person that is constantly looking outside themselves to see what needs to be done. If an older woman in front of you has dropped a package you be the person that jumps to pick it up for her. Get outside of your own grievances and complaints and begin to look at the world around you, there are a whole lot of people out here that need a whole lot of help.

It is so much easier to walk through the process of change when you are making your life about other people. I promise you that serving other people will bring you great joy and it will also help you move through the uncomfortable phases of your own changing.

"Who do I help?" you ask. Just open your eyes and look around you. Many people are living a miserable existence because they are so wrapped up in themselves and their own issues that they can't see their way clear to gratitude and happiness. When you are living a life that contributes to others, your own issues have a magical way of solving themselves.

Commit to the Process

Commitment does not take place where energies are scattered or dissipated. Therefore in order to be committed to your goals of change you must focus your energy and attention on the task at hand. Once you have your goals and your plans of action you must commit yourself to the process for better and for worse. Real commitment means that you stay with the process **NO MATTER WHAT**. It means that you keep going even when it's hard and you want to give up. It means that you keep going even when you are angry and uncomfortable. It means that you keep going even if it looks like there are no results. I am going to share with you the best piece of advice I have ever been given:

NEVER, EVER JUDGE ANYTHING BY THE WAY IT LOOKS. NEVER JUDGE BY THE CIRCUMSTANCES THAT APPEAR TO BE AROUND YOU. JUDGE A SITUATION ONLY BY YOUR INTENTION FOR THE OUTCOME.

This means that you tailor your thoughts, feelings and actions based only on what you intend for the outcome of a particular situation. For example: you are on a weight loss program and you have a bad day in which you gained three pounds. You simply acknowledge the information and move on, getting back on track and knowing that you are meeting your goals no matter what it looks like in the moment. <u>You do not</u> fall completely to pieces and spend the next three days stuffing your face because all is lost and you will be fat forever. Circumstances DO NOT dictate outcomes, intentions dictate outcomes.

There is an immense amount of power in staying committed to something no matter what. Toni Stone says it in a way that I love, she says…"simply stand in the middle of everything, anything…STAND THERE WITH INTENTION… don't get blown away by the storming going on around you…whether its about money, career, parents, relationships or paying the phone bill. STAND, KNOWING THAT WHAT'S BEEN DECLARED WILL BE THE CASE AS LONG AS YOU DON'T CHANGE YOUR MIND, DON'T WAVER, DON'T BACK DOWN EITHER, stand in…boots or ballet slippers, but stand…wear your cowboy hat or the flowered netting but don't slump at the wheel and whine."

Your commitment is your ability to stand in the face of anything/everything and know that things will turn out the way you've planned. You will stop smoking, you will leave that disempowering relationship, you will lose weight, you will get the perfect job and in the middle of getting to the goal it may look all kinds of different ways. The important point here is that you stand in the middle of your life intending for what you want and that you refuse to be moved in any other direction. Unpleasant circumstances quickly dissipate with lack of attention. Remember to speak only about what you want more of, as your words go forward to create your future.

If you can stay committed in the face of all your doubts you will see the circumstances alter to support your goals and intentions. Most people can't stay committed to any person or thing because they are easily swayed by appearances.

Practice Discipline

Webster's defines **discipline** as: *training that develops self-control, character, or orderliness and efficiency.* I define discipline as setting up and following a structure even when I don't like it. Discipline is one of those 'trigger' words for a lot of us, it brings to mind things like strict parents and military school. The truth is, without discipline nothing worthwhile would occur in our lives. The act of discipline is often the backbone of great happenings and certainly commitment cannot be practiced without discipline.

When we are faced with making changes in our behaviors and in our lives we must call on and enact the quality of discipline. Discipline puts the legs under our ideas for change. Discipline is doing the daily tasks over and over that support our goals and intentions for change. A disciplined person is one who does what they need to do no matter what the chatter in their head tells them. Your mind will run the gamut of excuses about why you don't need to get up early, eat right, exercise, be on time, drink enough water, get your work done, etc. Simply being disciplined enough to complete the tasks at hand will quell the chattering mind. Thank your mind for sharing and just move on to complete what needs to be done.

Everyday I have at least 12 excuses why today is not a good day to get on the treadmill for 30 minutes. The excuses vary from I don't feel like it to I'll do it later to I'm too busy or it's too hot in here. Any excuse seems like a good one. Everyday I listen to the chatter inside my head and I thank it for sharing and then I turn on the treadmill and start walking. I've found that the discipline of doing the treadmill in the morning before I do anything else works best for me. If I put it off it doesn't happen.

The more disciplined you become the more fine tuned your life will be, as there is an inner peace that establishes itself in a disciplined, action oriented person. Your worthiness index will go up when you are taking the actions you need to take in your life. When you feel good about yourself good things will find their way to you as like attracts like.

Surround Yourself with Supportive People

This is one of the most important aspects of any successful venture in life, surrounding yourself with the people that want to see you WIN and be a success. We have all kinds of people in our lives, the ones we help, the ones that help us, the ones we take care of, the ones we seek out for advice, the ones that are related, the ones that suck the life out of us, the ones that haven't changed, and the ones that are glad we are not winning because they are not winning. I have learned some very heartbreaking lessons when it comes to who you think supports you. As I have progressed in my process and my success in life has expanded there have been levels of people that have fallen away. This falling away has not been without heartbreak for me. I have had people that I thought were dear friends be very unkind to me as I became healthy and thin and they did not. The more I tried to encourage them to join me the meaner they became. Eventually I had to just accept that some people do not wish to change and I moved on. It takes a particular wisdom that comes from having your heart broken open to understand that people will do what they want and no matter how much we love them we cannot enact their changing. When you truly understand this, your life will become a lot simpler and you will recognize that the only person you can or need to control is YOU. This is a lesson I continue to learn everyday.

When you make the decision to move forward with changes in your life you will need to take a careful assessment of the people around you. Make sure that your desire to change is based on what YOU want for your life not what someone else thinks you should do. An example of this would be making sure that if you are married you decide to lose weight for you and your health, not because your spouse feels that you are overweight. Find the people in your life that support your ideas for change, most likely these will be the people that are already actively engaged in making the most of their own lives. Proactive people naturally attract to each other as people that feel victimized by life often wind up hanging out together. Like attracts like and you will naturally bring into your life the people that you require to forward your mission. Life itself will also naturally move you away from the people that inhibit your progress, sometimes this is the sad part. Remember that nothing is ever taken away that there isn't something better on its way. You have to have Faith. I do. The Universe will always send you a replacement for whatever you think you've lost, all you need to do is know it's on the way. Continue to affirm that your good is always on its way to you in whatever forms are best.

Don't be afraid to let go of the people, places or things that no longer suit you. If you clear out space in your life, the Universe will move quickly to provide you with the people, places and things that will support you. A support system that works is invaluable as these are the people that will remind you of your commitment when you have forgotten.

Focus on other people and what you can do for them, stay committed to your goals and practice the daily disciplines required to achieve them and surround yourself with people that really want you to WIN in life.

I know Jeff will have some good comments about this chapter...

And Jeff Says...

Every night when I go to bed, I replay the current day's events in my head. I ask myself:

How could I have improved myself today?
Did I spend enough time with my kids?
Did I eat healthy today?
Was I self-disciplined enough?

In the past when I had a bad day the circumstances would overwhelm me and I would become very negative. Now through my commitment and discipline I have trained myself to overcome unpleasant circumstances and get back on track quickly.

I truly believe that if you want something bad enough you will commit yourself to that something until it becomes a part of you. In other words you will begin to mentally picture yourself as having already achieved it.

The reason people fail is that they do not stay focused on their commitments.

Surround yourself with people that fail and you will create failure. Surround yourself with like-minded people and you will create a mindset of success.

Happy Words
are my Choice

*Affirmations taken from <u>Seasons of Prosperity</u>
by Toni Stone, <u>www.wonderworks.org</u>*

- Happy words describe a happy world.
- I am changing words in my life.
- The words I speak, say how I am...
- When I use new words, I create new life.
- Words make ways-of-being, they are my choice.
- I use words to say, my chosen ways of being.
- Vocabulary adjustments change the quality
  of my perceptions
- Disempowering words have left my sentences,
  I have replaced them with words of power
  and accomplishment.
- My choice of happy words develops a new level
  of satisfaction for me.
- I break out of unhappy habitual emotional states
  by altering word patterns. Everything changes.
- I give up language that intensifies negative emotions.
- Happy words change my emotional direction
  and feeling.
- What I say is what I am.
  I pay attention to words today.
- Today my word choices, direct life to avenues
  of happiness and contentment.

"The outer conditions of a person's life will always be found to reflect their inner beliefs."

— James Lane Allen

"Change the way you look at things, and the things you look at change."

— Wayne Dyer

The Sixth Way...
Reconstruct Your State of Mind

Imagine for a moment that we lived in a world where people actually understood that the words they speak go forward to create their future. In that world there would be very little complaining or negativity and how peaceful it would be. If you were to ask me what I thought was the most important lesson for you in this book my answer would be for you to fully understand that your words, thoughts, feelings and actions create your future.

What we spend our time thinking about, talking about, listening to, looking at, reading and watching all have great bearing on what is created in our lives. Understanding this gives us great power. If your current circumstances are unsatisfactory it is well within your reach to change them. All you need is a little reconstruction coaching.

HINT: If you think it, if you speak it~ IT WILL COME TO PASS.

Direct Your Thoughts

Start to direct your thoughts to what you want more of instead of spending time thinking about what you don't want more of. Stop complaining about the things that aren't working. You have to acknowledge the things that aren't working so that you can correct them; however, there is no need to complain to everyone about them as this will only create more of whatever the problem is. The first step in this process is to merely become conscious about the words that you are speaking. Are you grateful? Do you constantly complain? Are you always talking about what's wrong? Do you speak ill of others? Do you praise and acknowledge people? Do your words inspire people? Do your words hurt people?

Once you have a clear picture of the kind of talking you are doing you can take actions to alter it. Begin to sprinkle some gratitude into your speaking, talk about what went right for the day, make an effort to see the good in situations and speak about that. You have the ability to direct your life and your future by directing your thoughts. You can change your whole outlook on life by simply changing your speaking.

Fake It Till You Make It

In the beginning, doing linguistic surgery on yourself will be extremely uncomfortable as your thoughts will still be the same old moldy ones from the past and your new words will seem stupid. This is where you fake it till you make it. Feelings follow thought so direct thought -- direct feeling. After awhile your new thoughts will turn into new feelings. For instance, you will start to talk about how successful you are and pretty soon you will feel like a success and then the circumstances for you to become a success will materialize.

Remember the movie 'Field of Dreams' when Kevin Costner's character built the baseball field and he just kept saying it would work. Everyone thought he was crazy and he just kept right on saying it would work and it did. Real life is actually like that for those of us that understand Universal Principles. You begin by speaking what you intend and then you start moving into the thoughts, feelings and actions that will bring it into being. Lots of times in the middle of doing this you will appear to others as stupid and they may even feel sorry you are so committed to what they think is a pipe dream.

Think of all the success stories you have heard, they all started out as an idea that had no background of obviousness. Somebody had the thought and they backed it up with feelings and actions and they brought it into being. So can you.

An excellent way to push yourself into new thought patterns is to do affirmations. Find or write affirmations that talk about how you want your life to be and then spend a few minutes each day reading them. I have been doing affirmations since I was 12 years old and these days I spend 20-30 minutes a day doing them. I have included some of my favorites in this book. An affirmation is a statement that affirms what you want to have happen. As in:

- I am healthy.
- I am successful.
- I am losing weight everyday
- I am grateful.

- I leave behind old states of mind
- I create a future unlike the past

Saying or reading affirmations is a great way to re-train the mind into thinking things that will move you forward into a prosperous, healthy future.

A Little Gratitude Goes A Long Way

There are so many things to be grateful for and yet most people demonstrate very little gratitude for anything. Expressing gratitude is the quickest way to bring good into your life as what you praise naturally increases. In addition to changing your speaking and thinking, practicing gratitude is a required component for rejuvenating your life. The very act of gratitude is regenerative to the soul. For those of you that aren't sure what gratitude or being grateful actually mean here are Webster's definitions:

Gratitude: *A feeling of thankful appreciation for favors or benefits received; thankfulness*

Grateful: *Feeling or expressing gratitude; thankful; appreciative*

When you find yourself in a bad state of mind start mentally listing the things that you have to be grateful for and yes there is ALWAYS something to be grateful for. Taking the time to think about what you are thankful for instead of thinking about what you are suffering from will allow miracles to occur in your life.

I remind myself to practice gratitude daily by making a list every night of what I am grateful for. You can even be grateful for things in advance to help bring them into being. I was grateful daily for my weight loss long before it manifested itself. I keep a gratitude journal in my bedside table and I make myself write something in it every night. This is another discipline that I force myself to practice and there are days that I don't like this one either. On bad days I feel hard pressed to get to gratitude so on those days the list is short, however it is still there.

Practice some gratitude and I promise that your acts of thankfulness will return to bless you many times over. It is also a great idea to teach children the skills of being grateful as early as possible given that they are our future.

From the Inside Out

True and long lasting change will occur from the inside out and must begin as an idea. Once you have the idea of changing you begin to put a plan in place and the workable plan includes changes in thought patterns, speaking, surroundings, company that you keep, feelings that you have and behaviors that you practice. The first change occurs inside you as you begin to see yourself in the new way. As you see yourself newly you begin to speak and think differently which will cause you to take different actions. Inner behavior starts to change and as a result outer circumstances will follow suit.

It doesn't work to try and start change from the outside in. If you changed your outer circumstances without reconstructing your state of mind the changes wouldn't stick. You can only rejuvenate your life from the inside out as your current circumstances were brought on by your current state of mind. Therefore, if you want to change your current circumstances you must first change your current state of mind. Remember that creation occurs in the unseen (mind) and manifests itself into the seen (reality). In other words, whatever you are creating in your mind with your thoughts and feelings will bring itself into manifestation. If you think you are unworthy and poor you will create that. If you think and feel fat and unhealthy you will create that. If you have the power, why not just create yourself as a success? A fit and healthy success that is.

Some of these ideas may be new to you and may seem a little strange, however I promise you that they work when properly applied as I have been actively using them since I was 12 years old. I encourage you to do your own research and give them a try; it certainly can't hurt to be positive and grateful, right?

Next it's time to practice the fine art of letting go. First, a word from Jeff.

And Jeff Says...

My family and I bought our first home over 17 years ago on Cape Cod. It was located in a quaint village with mostly retirees and low to middle income families. After 7 years, I knew it was time for a change and in order to reconstruct my state of mind I took drastic measures which may not work for everyone. It works best for me when I push myself to take big risks so this is what I did...

After several months of searching I was able to purchase a building lot in an exclusive Cape Cod neighborhood. Although the land's price tag far exceeded my present financial circumstances, I was determined that I would build my family's home there and that I would create the means to do so.

Throughout this uncomfortable process I continually encountered my fears and doubts and I continually forced myself onward toward the goal. I knew I had to put myself in a neighborhood populated by successful people and this new home was being built next to CEO's, lottery winners and corporate executives.

9 months later there I was, a struggling entrepreneur, mowing my own lawn surrounded on all sides by the landscapers of my successful

neighbors. The important part is I was there in that neighborhood in a new home, I made it!

You can create change in many different ways and sometimes you just have to force yourself into it.

I wanted to be more successful, so I knew I had to surround myself with people that were winning in life.

You can apply this same type of concept to your own life. It will work.

Freely and Happily
I FORGIVE

Affirmations taken from <u>Seasons of Prosperity</u> by Toni Stone, <u>www.wonderworksstudio.org</u>

- I affirm and fully participate with life around me
- I forgive everyone and everything that has annoyed me
- I forgive the Universe for all its playful changes
- I hold onto nothing and no one in animosity anymore
- I forgive all those who seemed to disappoint me
- I forgive important, significant others who did what I didn't want them to do
- I forgive all close relations for what I say they are and what I say they aren't
- I forgive people for changing without asking me
- I forgive some people for showing up
- I forgive other people for not showing up
- I forgive all the people who broke their word
- I forgive all those who stay around for "no good reason"
- I forgive those who have passed out of present sight
- I forgive "too much" and "not enough"
- I forgive circumstances for appearing in ways I have assessed inappropriate
- I forgive Divine Order for not being "my" order
- I forgive all the events I judged that came at the "wrong" time
- I forgive all insects, animals, plants and weather conditions that did not immediately delight me
- Free and happy; I continuously forgive and am forgiven

When one whom I have benefited with great hope unreasonably hurts me, I will learn to view that person as an excellent Spiritual Guide.
—An Ancient Proclamation of Forgiveness from China

"For if you forgive others their trespasses, your heavenly Father will also forgive you; but if you do not forgive others, neither will your Father forgive your trespasses."
— Matthew 6:14-15

The Seventh Way...
Use the Power of Forgiveness

The Webster's definition of **forgive** is: *to give up resentment against or the desire to punish; to stop being angry with; to pardon; to give up all claim to punish.* My working definition of forgive for this chapter is to simply let go.

There are so many people out in the world that are holding onto so much yucky stuff—bad childhoods, terrible marriages/divorces, abuse of some sort, anger from some past wrong done to them, bad business deals, insults, injuries, etc. Every person holding onto something like this feels very strongly about it and should you try to pry it away from them they get very angry. It is their stuff and they want to keep it right where it is, what they fail to realize is that harboring those yucky feelings is sucking the life right out of them.

I have been actively working with forgiveness for several years now as I was holding onto some resentful feelings from the past. Over the last few years as I continued to move forward in my life it became apparent to me that there was something in the way of my progress. After some soul searching I discovered that I was still holding onto resentments and bad feelings toward people from my past. In my speaking I had forgiven them but in my heart I was still willing them to be different and therefore had not truly let go. I started doing some active work on forgiving these people and as a result a 25 year old impossible relationship was miraculously changed. This turn of events was something I never conceived as possible. The power of forgiveness is truly awe inspiring.

When we forgive (let go of) someone or something it doesn't mean that we are consenting to or forgetting what has transpired, it simply means that we are willing to get rid of the dead energy that the situation or relationship has placed on our lives. Holding onto animosity over someone or something doesn't really teach the other person anything it merely interferes with our own ability to manifest good in our lives. Harboring resentments and wishing ill on other people actually stops our own flow of good and can make us sick. People often hold grudges to "teach" the other person a lesson or to try and hurt the other person as they have been hurt. This kind of thinking only ends up hurting us, as we are the ones that actively carry around the bad energy which can cause us to be depressed, overeat, lose sleep or have anxiety.

The Choice Is Yours

In order to forgive someone we had to first decide to take offense from their words or actions. Whenever they did what they did we had a choice to take offense or to let the incident blow over. The choice in that moment was ours. Most people go along in life doing the best that they possibly can for who they are in the moment and often we get angry because their best is not our idea of what the best should be. We think that we would act very differently if we were them, however, we are not them and we don't really know how it feels to be them. It is very easy to be offended by others when we fail to consider what aspects of their lives effect their actions. It is easier to think about forgiving someone when we begin to really think about what their lives are like and what circumstances may be influencing their actions. Perhaps they don't even mean to hurt us, perhaps they are just going along doing the best that they can and they don't even recognize that their actions or words are hurtful.

How we react to something is always our choice. We can choose to be contributed to, insulted or offended. We can choose to take another's actions personally or we can choose to just let things flow over us. If your best friend doesn't call you back you can choose to be angry and offended and make it mean something about your friendship or you can choose to decide that maybe they are just so self-involved that calling you hasn't even crossed their mind. You decide, the choice is yours. The first choice puts a wedge in your friendship and the second allows you to let it go and go on with your life.

Watch Your Frame of Reference

You are not the same person that you were 5 years ago and neither is anyone else you know. Perhaps you are still relating to some people in your life based on how they were in the past. Your frame of reference for certain people could be based on what you knew of them 5, 10 or 15 years ago. This means that when they show up acting differently, you miss it because your frame of reference for them is ingrained in past perceptions. When we hold things against people they tend to remain forever trapped in our minds the way that they were when the hurt occurred. It may be easier to forgive them if we starting looking at whom they have become instead of who they were way back when. This happens a lot with family members, we tend to view them only as we knew them back in the day, who they are now doesn't even show up for us. We all have things in our pasts that we would do differently, imagine how we would feel if someone only judged us from the way we acted at 20.

It is always a good policy to investigate your frame of reference for the people in your life, perhaps some of them deserve a fresh perspective.

Nobody Wins the Blame Game

Blaming other people for circumstances in your life is never helpful nor will it take you any place you want to go. Nobody can win at the blame game. The only way to win in life is to take responsibility for your own destiny. Stop blaming the past and the people in it for what doesn't work in your life. Start having some new thoughts about the people and situations you need to forgive (let go of). Forgiveness doesn't mean that the hurtful behavior is excused or forgotten, it simply means that you stop allowing those incidents to control your life. Forgiveness can take place after you have experienced the necessary emotions associated with the incident. Once the initial anger, sadness, outrage, disappointment, etc. has been processed there is a space for forgiveness. You may need to express your feelings in a constructive way before you can allow the process of forgiveness (letting go) to take place. It is healthy to experience your emotions; it is not healthy to continue to carry around bad feelings for months and years. Process the events and then let them go.

Look for the Lesson

I am a firm believer in the statement 'everything happens for a reason' and I look at every uncomfortable situation in my life and try to see what it wants to teach me. Sometimes I see the lesson right away and sometimes I just have to trust that it's there and that I will see it eventually. I have learned some of my most valuable lessons from the people and situations that have distressed me the most. When you are open to the possibility of being contributed to by every event in your life the unpleasant events seem to go by faster.

I have also learned that one of the best ways to diffuse an attack is to apologize for something right in the middle of it. For instance, "I'm sorry that you feel I've insulted you", or "I'm sorry that you think I hurt you on purpose". People attack you because they want attention or they are unhappy with themselves. If someone attacks you in conversation and you do not respond or you apologize this will diffuse the situation. A person can only fight with you if you let them. You cannot argue with someone who refuses to be engaged by you.

I have been told that what we don't like about other people represents something that we don't like about ourselves. If this is true the first action would be to forgive ourselves for all the things that we find unacceptable. If we can forgive ourselves successfully then we can move ahead to start forgiving others. Truly, truly everyone is going along doing the best that they can for who they are—maybe it's time we stopped being so hard on ourselves and others.

Start with a List

The investigation into forgiveness can be started with a simple list of the people, places and things that you feel you need to forgive and that need to forgive you. Once you have this information written down you can start to think about how best to proceed with the act of letting go.

There are many excellent books that discuss forgiveness and I actually found two websites that have huge resources on forgiveness materials:

www.forgivenessweb.com
www.forgivenessday.com

I have also listed some books in my suggested reading list at the end of this book.

Everybody has something or someone to forgive and the act of letting go is very freeing to the self and to humanity as a whole. I encourage you to look at where the power of forgiveness might be useful in your life and I promise you that the results from the acts of forgiveness will be magical. Let's see what Jeff thinks about forgiveness and then we are on to the 8th Way which is creating the future…

And Jeff Says...

I'm grateful God has given me a vehicle to help others change their lives.

I care about helping others improve their quality of life and I strive to help every person that I can.

However, like others, I have often been hurt by those I've tried to help. In fact I've had more than my 'fair' share of pain and disappointments.

Forgiveness is a difficult practice and I've come to understand that all hurt and disappointment is not intentional. In order to allow yourself a clear path to success it is necessary to forgive others.

Expectancy for Life's Good

From *A Tonic for the Mind,* by Toni Stone
www.wonderworksstudio.org

Life has workability with it.
I am in life…with life…of life.

Life succeeds with me. I am grateful.
I am willing to be and have success…
Unfoldment of GOOD happens.
I count on life.

I SEE EVIDENCE THAT LIFE WORKS all around me now.
Symbols and signs of possibility are all around me now.
Change represents POSSIBILITY.

I recreate myself, in mind, as a creature-of-possibility
instead of an icon from the past…I talk like I expect the best.
I act like I already have the best.
I move to give the best.
I begin now to think and feel in new ways.
"How can I serve the future best?" This question opens up
further results and plans for good…
benefit comes from all that I do today.

There's UNLIMITED POTENTIAL FOR PROSPERITY…
Unlimited income is mine to claim.
As I move forward into the FUTURE,
I feel God's Grace at work.

The Amazing GRACE OF GOD strengthens and upholds me

and all the people around me.
Renewed, restored life is experienced by all.

Gratitude abounds…

Something Greater

from <u>Bridging the Gaps</u>, by Toni Stone
www.wonderworksstudio.org

- As I am willing to be more responsible for good,
  I draw GREATER GOOD into my life.

- I am here for GOOD PURPOSE, focused and clear.
  There is PLENTY of opportunity for me.

- I am in the appropriate place, right now.
- My life is GREATER and DEEPER than just about
  my own needs and desires.

- There are Divine appointments
  beyond everyday circumstances:

  - People to be helped
  - Cures to be applied
  - Healings to happen
  - Resources to recall
  - Bridges to be built
  - Information to reveal
  - Associations to be acquired
  - Commitments to be continued
  - Disciplines to be determined
  - Results to be produced
  - Boundaries to dissolve
  - Events to be celebrated
  - Cooperations to continue
  - Conclusions to draw
  - Possibilities to manifest
  - Contributions to be extended
  - Certainties to reinforce

The Life I Want and Wish

from Bridging the Gaps, by Toni Stone
www.wonderworksstudio.org

- New thoughts create new conditions. I am grateful.
- Endless possibilities are present for me.
- I am enjoying a happier, healthier
  more rewarding life today.
- I bring blessing to more others everywhere I am.
- I am functioning in productivity.

- Everywhere I go…I can help and I do.
- I get help everywhere… parking places, project
  assistance, checks in the mail, pivotal advice, goods and
  services…I always have what helps
  at the exact time it's necessary…
  WHAT'S REQUIRED IS PRESENT ALWAYS.

- I am continually overcoming limits.
- Challenges and problems are settled,
  satisfied, and resolved.

- People are always helping each other
  wherever I am, it happens.

- The life I want and wish is so available.
  I am capable of transmitting more light.
  I allow eternal light to shine through and into my life.
  The purpose for which I have been created
  is clear now.

- In higher service I give more and I am given more.
- I have an increasing attitude of gratitude.
  I can be so very grateful everyday.

- I am surrounded by the love of God.

"Imagination is the beginning of creation. You imagine what you desire, you will what you imagine and at last you create what you will."
— George Bernard Shaw

"Cherish your vision and your dreams as they are the children of your soul; the blueprints of your ultimate achievements."
— Napoleon Hill

The Eighth Way...
Possibilities Exist~Create the Future You Want

Possibilities exist everywhere, all the time we just need to learn to look for them. Some people see possibilities and other people see problems. Perception in life is everything as your perception has the power to change circumstance. If you want to create a future unlike the past then I suggest you start to look for and create possibility in your life. You have the ultimate power to determine how your life turns out, nobody is out there 'doing it' to you. You are 'doing it' to yourself with the words that you speak, the thoughts that you think and the actions that you take. Be a catalyst for change in your own life; be adventurous enough to start creating new experiences. Don't wait around for someone else to make you happy or for someone else to offer you an opportunity—get out there and create your own.

Begin by finding some new thoughts to think. Construct thoughts about how wonderful and successful your life is and talk about the experiences that you want more of.

Even if your life seems dreary to you right now, start writing goals and taking actions for the kind of future that you want to have. Stop wasting time feeling bad and sad about the current state of affairs and get into action to improve the circumstances.

Remember From Within, Out

Real changing has to occur from the inside out so get working on improving your current state of mind. Train yourself to spend the majority of time thinking and talking about what you want more of. Give little attention to the circumstances that are unsatisfactory. With lack of attention the undesirable fades away. Get up and get moving, do some form of exercise to help improve your physical condition and your state of mind. Get a little gratitude in your life and help other people to improve their lives. Quit sitting around sulking about how your life is turning out, this is not helping anyone. God helps those who help themselves so move out and start taking action. Declare your house a No Whining Zone and inform everyone that complaints are no longer welcome unless they are accompanied by a request or a promise. Stop letting people dump their negative stuff in your space. Strive to be positive and look for the good and when you are feeling foul just keep quiet, it will pass.

Tools to Support A Future Unlike the Past

There are some tools for change that I have found to be very useful and I believe that it will be helpful to share them with you. Any drive for change requires a disciplined practice and a solid commitment on your part to do what it takes. As change is very difficult it is often helpful to have some support materials available to you, the Self Talk Tape is one of these items.

A Self Talk Tape is an imaginative way to think and feel through to new ways of being. It is a tool to help you reprogram the thinking patterns of your subconscious mind. The subconscious mind carries out the instructions it is given. This is why your thoughts move forward to create your future. Your old ways of thinking are what have brought you to your present circumstances. In order to get new circumstances we need to develop new thoughts. An excellent way to program new thoughts and new ideas into your mind is to hear them over and over again in your own voice.

It is estimated that we have over 55,000 thoughts per day. So, if we spend 15 minutes a day or more listening to our own voice repeating new thoughts we make excellent progress on reprogramming the mind. A Self Talk Tape is a 15 minute recording of your own voice speaking affirmations about things that you want to have happen in your life. Before recording yourself it is a good idea to put a script together of what you want to say. You can focus on a particular issue like weight loss, business success or forgiveness.

Affirmations are not necessarily statements of outer fact, they are statements of potentiality and possibility...stated and repeated with feeling, they will inspire, motivate and move new action to occur. As we have discussed, words have an amazing power to bring about change. When making a Self Talk Tape keep the following in mind:

- Be personal
- Be positive
- Use the present tense
- Use action words
- Use feeling words
- Be realistic but stretch

- Phrase your affirmation as if
  it is already accomplished
- Too many words in a statement
  make it hard to listen to...be specific and short

Use your Self Talk Tape daily. You can record on a CD or on a tape and you can certainly listen to it more than once a day. Record 15 minutes of speaking and then just play it over and over while driving or doing things around the house. Good to listen to these while sleeping too, as that is when the subconscious mind is active.

A sample Self Talk Script
could look something like this:

- I am thinner and healthier now
- I eat only foods that support my goals
- I exercise daily
- I have plenty of energy
- I am moving ahead in life
- I create a future unlike the past
- I see possibility everywhere
- I see the good in all situations
- I am a problem solver
- I have plenty of money
- I am excited about my life
- Relationships that no longer serve me fall away

Over the years I have used the Self Talk Tape when I needed some help in having new thoughts or ideas about certain situations. This may seem like a silly thing to you; however, I promise that it works. Go ahead, give it a try.

The second tool that I have used is called an Image Book. An Image Book is a fun tool to help you visualize the new circumstances that you want to bring into your life. An Image Book is an 8-1/2 x 11 inch sticky page photo album with full page, clear plastic adhesive sheets. In the book you place full color pictures, words and phrases that represent the circumstances that you want to manifest. You can go through magazines and catalogs to collect pictures of the things that you wish to bring into being. When I first began my weight loss journey my Image Book was filled with pictures of thin women in groovy underwear and bathing suits, new workout clothes, new sneakers, people exercising and different words that affirmed weight loss and healthy ways of living.

Use colorful pictures and positive words and statements in creating your Image Book, a comprehensive book has between 50 and 100 pages and covers many aspects of your life: self-image, home, family, work, wealth, career, health and relationships. It is very important that you keep this type of book to yourself and only share it with others that are interested in the concept of creating one. There are some people that would demean this type of activity and they might even think that you couldn't possibly have what you are picturing for yourself. So keep what you are picturing for your future private.

Imagination is a primary power as imaging, feeling and thinking shape our life experiences. The Image Book helps open up new belief systems about ourselves, we begin to see ourselves as able to achieve what we want for the future. The pictures in the Image Book help us to dissolve old belief systems and replace them with new, more desirable ones. It is recommended that you look at your Image Book every night before you go to bed. Imagination creates new outcomes and you can construct new possibilities for yourself with regular use of the Image Book. As you look at the pages you will start to feel like the person you want to become. I have been using an Image Book since I was 12 years old and I continue to utilize this tool to create my future.

Exceed Expectations

It is time for you to go past where you want to stop in life; it's time to exceed your past expectations for the future. You can do and be anything that you want no matter how old you are. First, you must create the idea and then you must back it up with the thoughts, words, feelings and actions that will bring it into being. Remember, you and you alone possess the power to change your future. I suggest that you use that power to create something worthwhile for your life that will contribute to the lives of those around you.

Take a good long look at your life and decide what the areas are that require change. Get into action to change what needs to be changed so that you can jump out of bed excited about your life. Don't wait, DO IT NOW, start small if you have to, just as long as you start. You will feel so much better about yourself when you are doing the things that you need to do to make yourself happy and fulfilled. Don't concern yourself with what other people think and say about you, who cares? What matters is what you say about you. If you are living true, your spirit will automatically enliven and inspire others. People will want to know what you are doing and they will want to do it too.

The power belongs solely to you, use it wisely. Don't be afraid of hard work, it builds character. The time to change your life is now so get up and get moving— tomorrow is too... late...DO IT NOW.

*** Self Talk Tape** and **Image Book** description and instructions are adapted from Is Money the Matter: Chapter 8 by Toni Stone, www.wonderworksstudio.org*

And Jeff Says...

I have often said that to create success you must first envision it. The creative power of imagination is an extremely powerful tool and one that I use often.

When I first started out creating supplements I used to mock up product labels and tape them to vitamin bottles. Then I would place my 'new' products on the shelves in my office and envision how a customer would perceive them. When company came over I would proudly display the bottles in the kitchen and ask for opinions.

Although the process of first envisioning your success may require some creativity, it works. It is my suggestion that you start to use this method to help you reach your goals and make positive changes in your life.

I could talk forever about this chapter; however, I'm saving the rest of my thoughts for our upcoming book...CEO Makeover.

It is my intention that my insights at the end of each chapter will help you to make a Practical Change in your life.

I will see you on the road to success...

Epilogue

Well folks that's a wrap. My wish for you is that you are inspired to do something great with your lives, that somewhere in here you have recognized that you possess the skills to create the best possible future for yourself. Each of us has a unique gift to give and we need to get busy sharing those gifts with the people around us. As a culture we could stand to be happier, healthier and more grateful. As individuals we could stand to contribute more to other people and to stop complaining so much about what isn't working. We can all do more than what we are currently doing, there is always more to give.

I believe that it is of utmost importance to educate our children in matters of good health, gratitude and the fact that they possess the power to create incredible futures for themselves. To support this belief, Jeff and I have created the **Nature's Youth Fit Kids Foundation** which is a non-profit organization designed to offer educational programs to children. The educational programs offered will be based on the principles in this book and 5% of the gross profit from the Practical Change book and seminars will be donated to the Foundation.

I am deeply grateful to you for buying and reading this book and as I said at the beginning I intend that you have discovered something worthwhile in its pages.

If you are interested in having us come and do a PRACTICAL CHANGE seminar for your business, please feel free to ask us for more information.

We wish for you the most blessed future and we welcome your comments or questions in regard to this material.

Please feel free to contact us at:

Noelle@naturesyouth.com
jjones@naturesyouth.com

or via mail at

Noelle Federico or
Jeff Jones
Nature's Youth, Inc.
1616 Westgate Circle
Brentwood, TN 37027

Also please be sure to visit us at
www.naturesyouth.com and
www.practicalchanges.com

Thank You and God Bless!

Noelle and Jeff

PRACTICAL CHANGE –

Sources

Websites:

www.americanheart.org
www.hsph.harvard.edu/nutritionsource/index.html
www.iom.edu
www.health.gov/dietaryguidelines
www.glycemicindex.com
www.ama-assn.org

Publications:

Nutrition Action Health Letter
September 2004, Volume 31/Number 7

Books:

The Everything Total Fitness Book:
A complete program to help you look and feel great
by Ellen Karpay,
Adams Media Corporation, Avon, MA, 2000.

Seasons of Prosperity:
An Intentional Prayer Book
by Toni Stone
Wonderworks Studio, Fairfax, VT, 1996.

Is Money the Matter - Chapter Eight:
Even Parking Lots Have Blueprints
by Toni Stone
WonderworksStudio, Fairfax, VT, 2003.

A Tonic for the Mind:
Affirmations for Every Kind of Day
by Toni Stone
Wonderworks Studio, Fairfax, VT, 2003.

The Nature's Youth Product Line

I have provided a list of our products along with a brief description. For more detailed information, pricing and supplemental facts please visit **www.naturesyouth.com**

Nature's Youth RSF

An amino acid precursor that helps the body naturally increase its levels of the Human Growth Hormone. Our flagship anti-aging product can also help the body to lose fat and increase lean muscle mass. It was a HUGE help in my weight loss program.

Diet Lift (my favorite)

An ephedra-free appetite suppressant and energy enhancer that contains
~Citrus Aurantium
~ Green Tea
~ Guarana
~ Triple ginseng blend
(Panax ginseng, American ginseng, and Siberian ginseng)
~ Ginko Biloba
this product has helped me immensely.

Daily Defense (for Men or Women)

Our comprehensive Multi-vitamin that contains vitamins, minerals and digestive enzymes as well as support nutrients for men and women in different formulations.

Youthful Greens

Our green food supplement that will help make sure that you are getting the required amounts of fruits and vegetables in your daily diet. A must have addition to a good health regimen.

R-Factors

Our breakthrough anti-aging complex that contains Resveratrol. R-Factors is a major breakthrough in the field of age management. This all-natural formula addresses the most critical biological processes associated with aging. Most researchers agree that the 3 primary factors to influence aging are; oxidation (free radical damage), glycation (elevated blood sugar and insulin levels) and caloric consumption. R-Factors is the first and only age management formula to address these 3 primary factors of aging. This is an excellent companion product to Nature's Youth RSF.

Cal Defense

An effervescent Calcium/Magnesium supplement. The calcium in Cal Defense can help strengthen bones, while the magnesium can relieve tension and aid in relaxation. Cal Defense has a unique delivery system that offers maximum absorption. As a drink, Cal Defense enters your system as a liquid, and is broken down before it reaches the stomach. Just mix it with cold water, and you won't have to swallow all those pills to get the calcium you need.

Coral Blend

A Coral Calcium supplement formulated from Sea Coral. Sea coral provides high concentrations of calcium, along with dozens of other minerals that occur naturally in the environment.

Red Stag for Men

An all natural testosterone booster for men. Red Stag is formulated with some of the most frequently studied natural ingredients that are shown to increase testosterone levels. Increased testosterone levels have been known to increase sex drive as well as reduce body fat, increase lean muscle mass and improve energy.

Nature's Youth Noni Juice
(I swear by this stuff and take it daily)

- Our Noni is 100% Tahitian Noni and is not reconstituted.
- Boosts general health and performance
- Dramatic improvement in weakened conditions
- Increases absorption and utilization of vitamins, herbs and minerals
  (the food and other supplements in your diet)
- Powerful antioxidant function— protection from free radical damage
- "The sacred fruit for regenerating the body"
- A staple of nutritional supplement program
  — to be taken daily

Noni fruit has been used for over 2,000 years. Ancient medicine men used it as their most important health remedy. Today, substantial research has led scientists to validate Noni's unique healing benefits. Noni is documented to be effective against bacteria (including E. coli), have unique immune stimulating effects, and contain many phytonutrients and enzymes (including proxeronine) related to healing. As an adaptogen, Noni helps maintain balance of the body's organs through regulation of cellular function, acting where most needed in the body.

Carb Buster
Carb-Buster is an amazing, non-stimulant, all-natural nutritional supplement derived from the white kidney bean. It contains Phase 2 (r), the first nutritional ingredient clinically proven to neutralize starch. It is the starch in your favorite foods that contribute to weight gain.

Enerox

A powerful energy anti-oxidant formula. In addition to providing exceptional antioxidant support Enerox is formulated with Green Tea and Seville Orange biflavonoids to provide you with extra energy. Green Tea is known for its ability to provide extra energy as well as anti-oxidant support. Green Tea is a natural source of caffeine that gives you that extra boost needed to make it through the day.

Youth Flex (another of my favorites, this stuff is great)
A Powerful Joint Support Formula with IsoOxygene™ and Glucosamine

- Formulated to Sooth Joint Stress and Sore Muscles
- 500 mg of IsoOxygene™
- 500 mg of Glucosamine Sulfate for Added Joint Support
- 200 mg of Cetyl Myristoleate to help lubricate joints and connective tissue
- 50 mg of Boswellia Serrata gum extract to help improve blood supply, shrink inflamed tissue and reduce stiffness

PRACTICAL CHANGE –

Nature's Youth Product Coupon

If you would like to try any of our products you may order them online at **www.naturesyouth.com** or call us at 800~333~6923

Please use coupon code:
Practical Change
to receive 20% off your order.

Thank you for your interest in our products, **Nature's Youth** is committed to promoting Good Health.

Noelle's Suggested Reading List

The Positive Principle Today
by Norman Vincent Peale

The Power of Positive Thinking
by Norman Vincent Peale

Think and Grow Rich by Napoleon Hill

The Dynamic Laws of Prosperity
by Catherine Ponder

Science and Health: With Key to the Scriptures
by Mary Baker Eddy

The Millionaires of Genesis by Catherine Ponder

The Secret Door to Success
by Florence Scovel Shinn

Your Best Life Now:
7 Steps to Living at Your Full Potential
by Joel Osteen

The Prospering Power of Love by Catherine Ponder

Food Politics by Marion Nestle

The 7 Habits of Highly Effective People: Powerful Lessons in Personal Change
by Stephen R. Covey

The Power of Now:
A Guide to Spiritual Enlightenment
by Eckhart Tolle

The Science of Mind:
A Philosophy, A Faith, A Way of Life
by Ernest Holmes

Every Saint Has A Past, Every Sinner A Future:
Seven Steps to the Spiritual
and Material Riches of Life
by Terry Cole-Whittaker

The Perricone Promise:
Look Younger, Live Longer in Three Easy Steps
by Nicholas Perricone, M.D.

Weight Loss That Lasts:
Breakthrough the 10 Big Diet Myths
by James M. Rippe, M.D. and Weight Watchers

The 3-Hour Diet by Jorge Cruise

8 Minutes in the Morning by Jorge Cruise

Fat Land: How Americans Became
the Fattest People in the World by Greg Crister

Fast Food Nation by Eric Schlosser

Shrink Your Female Fat Zones by Denise Austin

Seasons of Prosperity by Toni Stone

Is Money the Matter by Toni Stone

A Tonic for the Mind by Toni Stone

Heal Your Life by Louise Hay